# WordTOOLS For Self Esteem

Vol. 2

Harnessing the
Power of Words!

Carol L Rickard, LCSW

Well YOUniversity® Publications

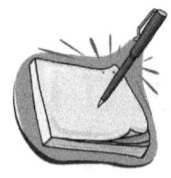

**Sign up now!**

To be sure to get our weekly motivational & inspirational quotes and stories!

**ThePowerOfWordsEQuote.com**

Copyright © 2017 Carol L. Rickard

All Licensing by Well YOUniversity, LLC

All rights reserved.

ISBN-13: 978-1-947745-07-0

# WordTools for Self Esteem Vol. 2
## Harnessing the Power of Words!
by Carol L Rickard, LCSW

© Copyright 2017 Well YOUniversity Publications

ISBN 13: 978-1-947745-07-0

All rights reserved.

No part of this book may be reproduced for resale, redistribution, or any other purposes (including but not limited to eBooks, pamphlets, articles, video or audiotapes, & handouts or slides for lectures or workshops).

Licenses to reproduce these materials for those and any other purposes must be obtained from the author and Well YOUniversity.

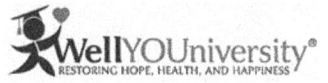

**888 LIFE TOOLS** (543-3866)

Carol@WellYOUniversity.com

# Welcome!

My 1st WordTool came to me in 2006 when doing a group with my patients. How could I get them to w*elcome* change in their lives?

**C**reating **H**ealthy **A**nd **N**ew **G**rowth **E**xperiences!

From there it's been an onward journey! Most of them are inspired by persons or situations. All of them I use in my own life. My hope is to create Ah-Ah moments that can help change a life!

They are officially called "Artinyms", which is Sanskrit for "describe".

On the back of each wordtool is a question for you. Answering them will serve to strengthen and build your self-esteem from the inside out!

~To Living Well TODAY! ~

Carol

| | | | | |
|---|---|---|---|---|
| ACT | 1 | IMAGINE | 31 |
| ADAPT | 3 | INTENTIONS | 33 |
| ATTITUDE | 5 | MIND | 35 |
| BASE | 7 | NEEDS | 37 |
| CHANGE | 9 | NOTICE | 39 |
| COMPLAIN | 11 | PAIN | 41 |
| COPE | 13 | PATIENCE | 43 |
| DOING | 15 | POWER | 45 |
| EGO | 17 | START | 47 |
| FEAR | 19 | STRESS | 49 |
| FOCUS | 21 | THRIVE | 51 |
| GOALS | 23 | TODAY | 53 |
| GUILT | 25 | TRY | 55 |
| HEALING | 27 | VOICE | 57 |
| HOPE | 29 | WANTS | 59 |

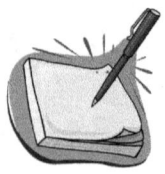

**Sign up now!**

To be sure to get our weekly motivational & inspirational quotes and stories!

**ThePowerOfWordsEQuote.com**

**A**cquire

**C**oping

**T**ools

COPYRIGHT 2017 & Licensed by Well YOUniversity, LLC

What is a situation you need to *act* on now in order to make your self-esteem stronger?

**A**

**D**eliberate

**A**djustment

**P**roviding

**T**ransformation

COPYRIGHT 2017 & Licensed by Well YOUniversity, LLC

When is a time you *adapted* and how did it impact on your self-esteem?

**A**djusting

**T**hinking

**T**o

**I**ntentionally

**T**ake

**U**s

**D**irection

**E**xcellence

COPYRIGHT 2017 & Licensed by Well YOUniversity, LLC

How would you describe your *attitude*? Does it need adjusting? Is it helping or hurting your self-esteem?

**B**uilding

**A**

**S**olid

**E**xistence

COPYRIGHT 2017 & Licensed by Well YOUniversity, LLC

What are the things you need present in your life to have a strong *base*?

**C**reating

**H**ealthy

**A**nd

**N**ew

**G**rowth

**E**xperiences

COPYRIGHT 2017 & Licensed by Well YOUniversity, LLC

What are some important *changes* you could make in your life that would pay off BIG?

**C**oncentrate

**O**n

**M**aking

**P**roblems

**L**arger

**A**ctually

**I**ncreasing

**N**egativity

COPYRIGHT 2017 & Licensed by Well YOUniversity, LLC

What are some of the things you tend to **complain** about? What can you do instead?

**C**hallenge

**O**ur

**P**roblems

**E**ffectively

COPYRIGHT 2017 & Licensed by Well YOUniversity, LLC

What are some of your healthy *coping* tools? Are there areas you need to get better at, if so, what?

**D**irect

**O**pportunity &

**I**ncrease

**N**et

**G**rowth

COPYRIGHT 2017 & Licensed by Well YOUniversity, LLC

What is something you have started *doing* that is making a + difference on your self-esteem?

**E**stablishes

**G**reat

**O**bstacles

COPYRIGHT 2017 & Licensed by Well YOUniversity, LLC

How have *you* gotten in the way of yourself and what was the impact on your self-esteem?

**F**ind

**E**motion

**A**lters

**R**eality

COPYRIGHT 2017 & Licensed by Well YOUniversity, LLC

What has **fear** stopped you from doing? How do you think this has impacted on your self-esteem?

**F**ix
**O**ur
**C**oncentration
**U**ntil
**S**uccessful

COPYRIGHT 2017 & Licensed by Well YOUniversity, LLC

What areas can you *focus* on that will help strengthen your self-esteem?

**G**etting

**O**ur

**A**ctivities

**L**ined-up

**S**traight

COPYRIGHT 2017 & Licensed by Well YOUniversity, LLC

Do you already have *goals* set for yourself? If so, what are they? If not, why not?

**G**rieve

**U**nresolved

**I**ncidents

**L**imiting

**T**oday

COPYRIGHT 2017 & Licensed by Well YOUniversity, LLC

Do you struggle at all with *guilt*? What are some things you feel that way about? Why?

**H**olding

**E**motion

**A**nd

**L**etting

**I**t

**N**aturally

**G**o

COPYRIGHT 2017 & Licensed by Well YOUniversity, LLC

What are some of the experiences in your life where **healing** still needs to take place?

**H**olding

**O**nto

**P**ositive

**E**xpectations

COPYRIGHT 2017 & Licensed by Well YOUniversity, LLC

If you could have *hope* things would get better, what would change in your life?

**I**ncredible

**M**ental

**A**ctivity

**G**enerating

**I**deas

**N**ot

**E**xisting!

COPYRIGHT 2017 & Licensed by Well YOUniversity, LLC

If you were to let yourself *imagine* things being different in your life – what changes could you see?

**I**nvisible

**N**ergy

**T**hat's

**E**xtended &

**N**ecessary

**T**o

**I**nviting

**O**pportunities

**N**eeded

**S**ucceed

COPYRIGHT 2017 & Licensed by Well YOUniversity, LLC

How do you think your *intentions* are impacting on your self-esteem?

**M**agical

**I**nstrument

**N**eeding

**D**irection

COPYRIGHT 2017 & Licensed by Well YOUniversity, LLC

What are the instances where you weren't paying attention & made some unhealthy decisions?

**N**ecessary

**E**lements

**E**nabling

**D**aily

**S**urvival

COPYRIGHT 2017 & Licensed by Well YOUniversity, LLC

What are some of your *needs* when it comes to growing your self –esteem?

**N**atural

**O**pportunity

**T**o

**I**nspect

**C**urrent

**E**xperiences

COPYRIGHT 2017 & Licensed by Well YOUniversity, LLC

For the next 24 hours, *notice* what goes on during your day & come back to write about it!

**P**owerful

**A**lignment

**I**nfluencing

**N**egativity

COPYRIGHT 2017 & Licensed by Well YOUniversity, LLC

Did you know the more your focus on *pain* the stronger it gets? Instead, focus on relief! What has pain stopped you from doing?

**P**ut

**A**side

**T**ime

**I**nstead

**E**ngage &

**N**otice

**C**urrent

**E**nvironment

COPYRIGHT 2017 & Licensed by Well YOUniversity, LLC

Think of a time when you had ***patience***. How did that impact your self-esteem? Now think of a time when you had none – How did that impact?

**P**utting

**O**urselves

**W**here

**E**xcellence

**R**esults

COPYRIGHT 2017 & Licensed by Well YOUniversity, LLC

What are some places where you can connect to *power*? Are there people who can connect you?

**S**wiftly

**T**ake

**A**ction

**R**eaching

**T**argets

COPYRIGHT 2017 & Licensed by Well YOUniversity, LLC

What are some behaviors you need to *start* doing in order to strengthen your self-esteem?

**S**teals

**T**he

**R**esources &

**E**nergy

**S**abotaging

**S**uccess

COPYRIGHT 2017 & Licensed by Well YOUniversity, LLC

What are some of your sources of **stress**?
What can you do to reduce your daily stress?

**T**o

**H**ave

**R**eached

**I**ncredibly

**V**alued

**E**xistence

COPYRIGHT 2017 & Licensed by Well YOUniversity, LLC

How do you honestly feel about yourself? Can you identify any strengths you value? What strengths do others think you have?

**T**he
**O**nly
**D**ay
**A**fforded
**Y**ou!

COPYRIGHT 2017 & Licensed by Well YOUniversity, LLC

How would your life and self-esteem be different if you were to only live in **today**? Do you ever find yourself getting lost in the past or the future?

**T**ake

**R**esponsibility

**Y**ourself!

COPYRIGHT 2017 & Licensed by Well YOUniversity, LLC

What are you willing to *try* that you have never been willing to do before?

**V**aluable

**O**pportunity

**I**nfluencing

**C**ircumstances

**E**veryday

COPYRIGHT 2017 & Licensed by Well YOUniversity, LLC

What some positive ways you can use your *voice* to stand up or help out someone else?

**W**ishful

**A**ctivities

**N**ot

**T**ied

**S**urvival

COPYRIGHT 2017 & Licensed by Well YOUniversity, LLC

What are the **wants** you have that could be preventing your self-esteem from growing? What would it be like to let them go?

## About the Author

Carol L Rickard, LCSW, TTS, of Hopewell, NJ is founder & CEO of WellYOUniversity, LLC, a global health education company dedicated *to empowering individuals with the tools and supports to achieve lifelong wellness & recovery.*

Also known as **America's Wellness Ambassador**, Carol is a dynamic & engaging speaker who brings to life practical / useful solutions. She is a weekly contributor for Esperanza Magazine; written 13 books on stress and wellness, had a guest appearance on Dr. Oz last year

She is also the creator & host of a 30-minute wellness show on Princeton TV - **The WELL YOU Show** which current episodes are aired on Mondays at 6:00pm EST & Sundays at 8:30am EST and can be watched at PrincetonTV.org.

All episodes available at: **www.TheWELLYOUShow.com**

Get more of Carol at:

Twitter: ***@wellYOUlife***

"Like us" @ www.FaceBook.com/WellYOUniversity

# Have Carol Speak at Your Next Event!

Get more information about how you can have Carol speak at your organization, event, or conference.

Go to: www.CarolLRickard.com

Or call: 888 Life Tools (543-3866)

### Carol's Other Books

*Getting Your Mind to Mind You*
*ANGER – A Simple & Practical Approach*
*Help – How to Help Those Who DON'T Want it*
*Selfness – Simple Self-Care Secrets*
*Stress Eating – How to STOP Using Food to Cope*
*Stretched Not Broken – Caregiver's Stress*
*The Caregiver's Toolbox*
*Transforming Illness to Wellness*
*Putting Your Weight Loss on Auto*
*The Benefits of Smoking*
*Moving Beyond Depression*
*LifeTools – How to Manage Life*
*Creating Compliance*
*Relapse Prevention*

**Please visit us at:**

**www.WellYOUniversity.com**

Sign up for weekly motivational e-quote!

Check out our upcoming FREE webinars!

Learn more about our training programs.

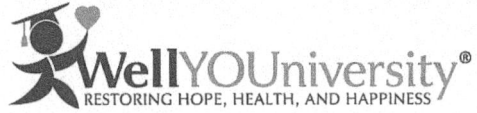

Email us your success story at:

Success@WellYOUniversity.com

*We'd like to ask for your feedback*

Please check out the next page
if this book has been HELPFUL for you!

## We'd love to hear from you!

### Feedback Card

Please take a moment & provide us some feedback about the book you just read & how you feel *it benefited YOU!*

_____

_____

_____

_____

Tear along here

Name: _____

Best Phone #: _____

Can we use your comments in our publicity materials?

Yes / No

If OK with you, what's the best time to call you:_____

Thank You!

**Scan or take a picture & email:**
Carol@WellYOUniversity.com

**Snail mail:** Carol Rickard
5 Zion Rd., Hopewell, NJ 08535

www.ingramcontent.com/pod-product-compliance
Lightning Source LLC
LaVergne TN
LVHW051209080426
835512LV00019B/3176